Foot Reflexology

The Ultimate Foot Reflexology Guide

James Heath

Table Of Contents

Introduction

Whether it's about going on a usual errand or standing for hours at work, your feet have to bear with all kinds of pressure, tension and trouble all the time.

But, do you ever give this important body part a chance to breathe? Have you ever considered relaxing your feet to release the tension that has built up over the years?

Did any tell you that you can become more energetic, healthy and active by seeking the help of foot reflexology?

From healing your tired heels to relaxing the tiny tips of your toes, foot reflexology is an excellent wellness approach that relies on scientific principles to care for your feet.

From addressing circulatory issues, sports injuries, heal spurs to taking care of the diabetic foot, this art of foot reflexology offers countless healing benefits to your feet.

As they say, "The foundation of a tree depends on its roots, and the stronger the roots, the stronger the tree". Similarly, the healthier your feet, the healthier your body. By employing the most effective natural oils to relax your feet, foot reflexology heals your body, mind and soul.

A Bit About The Background

Ancient forms of medicine and massage have been recognized nowadays by experts with their proven healing capabilities. The Chinese, Egyptians, Indians and others have all practiced the so-called method of reflexology.

But what exactly is it and how does it benefit your overall health?

First of all, reflexology is a special form of massage. It doesn't just relax a certain part of the body that's the target of the massage, but it also sends the pressure towards the other body parts.

Some people may also target the hands but it's usually done through the foot, hence, people call it "foot reflexology".

Most of us nowadays are bent on working long hours, with almost little or no time to have ourselves checked and relaxed. The power of reflexology helps us attain our desired health through a series of pressurized massages to relieve certain pain.

This technique is mostly enjoyed by adults and elders who experience body and joint pains most of the time.

The Real Benefits of Foot Reflexology

Much like oriental and herbal medicine, as well as acupuncture, it is no doubt that people are embracing the painless way of healing through therapeutic massage. To explain more of its good sides, here are the great health benefits of foot reflexology:

Improved Blood Circulation

Perhaps you have heard it – and yes, you're right. The blood circulation of a person is improved through this type of foot massage because the gentle and accurate strokes of the feet can trigger normal and distributed blood flow.

Uric acid and similar stuff can accumulate in our bloodstream, which can possibly cause certain illnesses and diseases. Gravity further pushes it downwards to the feet.

To prevent this from happening, reflexology techniques are applied to evenly distribute the blood flow and keep it constant. It can also distribute nutrients to other parts of the body faster. Indeed, foot reflexology is a good way to keep our system up and running.

Pain Reduction Through Endorphin

Endorphins are stronger elements than morphine as a painkiller – meaning they can block certain instances of pain and thereby relax the patient. Through reflexology techniques, one can have reduced pain through the stimulation of endorphin through the foot massage and pressures.

One of the most common examples of pain that reflexology techniques can cure is the PMS or premenstrual syndrome for women, soothing the reproductive system – it involves certain pressure points around the ankle and the big toe.

The Advantage of Relaxation

With the help of foot reflexology, you can feel

more relaxed and far away from stress, depression and other negative mental states. In terms of reflexology, there are numerous reflex points, which can have significant benefits on the patient.

One such is the solar plexus, which stores the person's stress. Reflexology helps release these stress hormones, since stress can have bad effects to the immune system as well.

Improve Channels

The Chinese experts believe that reflexology can balance a person's Yin and Yang by maintaining the channels at the feet. If you're familiar with Meridian points in acupuncture, then you might get a better idea of foot reflexology concepts.

According to them, if these channel points become blocked, it causes pain and stress to certain parts of the body, so the main objective of reflexology techniques is to unblock these channel points and restore a patient's health.

Memory Enhancement

If you are having trouble remembering things due to age or some other reason, then you might need to undergo reflexology. It is said that a person's memory can be enhanced due to balancing the oxygen circulation in the blood.

Oxygen, an important component of the body, goes to the brain and improves its processing and storing of information. Foot reflexology, in short, is a helping tool for those who experience certain memory loss and forgetfulness.

Erogenous Stimulation and Relationship Building

For couples who are having problems with their sex life, foot massages and therapies can help with some erogenous stimulation, along with the relaxation and removal of stress.

Doing reflexology to each other not only helps improve your lovemaking skills, but also tightens the bond of any husband and wife. This is mostly because the feet have a lot of nerve endings and reflex points – great for sensual activity.

Reduces Anxiety and Depression

One of the best benefits of foot reflexology is shaking the stress away. When a person becomes stress-free, there is a lesser chance of developing anxiety disorders and depression.

So if you have a friend, family member or colleague who is undergoing real tough times, help him/her relax through the power of reflexology and feel better.

Good for Blood Pressure

If you are a person who is prone to getting high blood pressure, then a foot therapy session might help lower it down. It does not matter if your high blood pressure may be caused by genetic faults or imbalanced lifestyle – a good massage through the power of foot reflexology gives you a lower blood pressure.

Helps Cure Migraine and Headache

Still connected to the anti-stress benefits of reflexology, it helps cure headache and migraine, due to its painkilling properties. This has been proved in a Danish study, where 65%

of the respondents have reduced symptoms of migraine and headaches after undergoing reflexology sessions, without the help of medications.

Good for Pregnant Women

Most pregnant women experience fluid retention in certain areas of the feet, also called edema. Regular massage therapy techniques can help reduce the swelling. It may also help in post-natal depression and menopause.

Good for Flat Feet

Foot reflexology is a beneficial therapy for

people with flat feet. It may also reduce and help in curing plantar fasciitis or the inflammation of certain foot tissue, which is usually experienced by people with flat feet.

Helps in Post-Operation Recovery

Due to its painkilling and relaxation properties, reflexology can help patients who have just undergone operation or surgery. Through this, the use of analgesics can be reduced.

Helps in Chemotherapy

Cancer patients who undergo reflexology also

have lesser side effects and helps reduce anxiety.

Understanding The Basic Meridians Found in Your Feet

In reflexology, the concept of meridians is the most basic thing to learn. Meridians are the certain points in the body that when applied therapeutic massage through reflexology techniques, can stimulate pressure that goes through certain parts of the body and help cure diseases.

In our body, there a total of 12 pathways by which energy can flow freely if opened through the techniques used in reflexology massage, and can cause their target organs to feel better.

These 12 pathways called meridians can be found on the hands and feet, but in this book, we will focus on understanding the basic meridians found in feet, starting with the most important concepts.

Meridian Congestion

Reflexology is a well-researched and proven science of healing. In the basic sense, meridian congestion refers to the blockage experienced by these pathways that may cause pain to different parts of the body. The energy called 'Chi' is the flowing energy that goes through these pathways (you've probably heard of it on Chinese medicinal concepts).

It is said that the blockage of these pathways

due to poor diet and health practices can lower the flourish of Chi in our body and eventually give way to diseases.

Thus, knowledge of basic meridians in our body is important to prevent meridian congestion to happen and improve our health.

Liver Meridian

The liver meridian is located at the big toe and connects to the liver of the person. It runs through the body, passing the gall bladder, legs and chest. In Chinese concepts, the wood element is the association of this meridian and classified as a yin pathway.

Our liver is a very important part of our body because it helps us detoxify our foods. It plays a big game in digestion, protein synthesis and metabolism of a person.

This is one of the basic meridians that when blocked or disturbed, can cause a number of disorders such as liver problems, fatigue, mental problems, abdominal and lower back pain and extreme anger or stress.

Stomach Meridian

The stomach meridian can be accessed from the foot's second toe (from the largest), but starts with the eye and branches down to the foot, passing the spleen and connects to the stomach. In Chinese concepts, the earth element is the association of this meridian and classified as a yang pathway.

Stomach pains are one of the usual hindrances of our health, depending on our diet. As one of the basic meridians, the stomach meridian also works with the spleen meridian.

The stomach is the key organ of food digestion, so when the stomach meridian does not function properly, any of the following health problems may arise: vomiting, abdominal problems, bloating and even mental problems.

It is also said that the stomach meridian can affect a lot of our body parts, since it passes through a lot of important internal organs.

Kidney Meridian

The kidney meridian is located on the sole of the foot and extending to the legs, bladder area and to the kidney and to the clavicle. One of the basic meridians, it works hand-in-hand with the gall bladder meridian.

In Chinese concepts, the water element is the association of this meridian and classified as a yin pathway.

Kidneys play a very important role in our body. It filters blood, helps keep our urinary system in shape and removes all other waste products that are left behind by metabolism.

Different problems may occur if the kidney meridian is blocked, such as some of the most expensive and life-threatening diseases of the kidney include kidney stones, kidney failure and urinary problems.

Gall Bladder Meridian

The gall bladder meridian is one of the basic meridians that starts with the eyes, like the liver meridian and stomach, can be accessed from the foot's second toe (from the largest). In Chinese concepts, the wood element is the association of this meridian and classified as a yang pathway.

Unlike the other meridian organs, the gall bladder can be safely removed from a person through cholecystectomy and survive normally.

However, blockage and damage to the gall bladder meridian may induce different kinds of pain to the ears, eyes, jaws, throat, and lower limbs and may also cause neuralgia (stinging pain from damaged nerves).

It is also one of the basic meridians associated with headache and eye problems. It may also cause pain in the teeth.

Urinary Bladder Meridian

The urinary bladder meridian, or simply bladder meridian, also starts from the eyes and going down to the little toe, passing by the neck, kidney, urinary bladder, buttocks and to the feet. In Chinese concepts, the water element is the association of this meridian and classified as a yang pathway.

As a very important organ in our body, the urinary bladder's overall health may be compromised when the urinary bladder meridian gets blocked with unhealthy habits or instances.

Just like all of the basic meridians, its blockage can cause illnesses, diseases and affect a number of organs and parts of our body including the urinary system and lower limbs. It may also be associated with eczema, headaches, mental problems and rheumatic pains.

Spleen or Pancreas Meridian

Last, but not the least, the spleen meridian, which is sometimes known as the pancreas meridian, lies at the big toe (next to the liver meridian's opening) and goes through the shoulders, passing by the legs, pelvis, abdomen, stomach, throat, liver and connects to the spleen. It also connects with the heart meridian.

And just like all of the basic meridians, it also has an associated element – earth, and is classified as a yin pathway.

The spleen meridian directly affects the spleen and pancreas, which work together with the stomach as internal organs and as meridians.

The spleen is responsible for iron circulation, holds stored blood, circulates and reorganizes red blood cells and metabolizes hemoglobin.

The spleen is important in preventing circulatory shock due to lack of oxygen. Blockage of the spleen meridian may result in vomiting, bloating, stomach problems and various anxiety disorders.

How to Perform Foot Reflexology Yourself

In the field of reflexology, much like in Chinese acupuncture, and as proven by scientists and health experts, the feet hold the key points called channels or meridians that, when applied proper pressure and massaging techniques, can have the ability to revitalize, relax and soothe our internal organs, external parts and other points of pain.

Nowadays, more and more people are switching to a more convenient, cheaper and practical way of healing with less usage for medications. This is where reflexology comes in handy.

If you have enough time and patience, here are some guidelines on how to correctly perform foot reflexology by yourself to anyone, or even yourself.

Understand the Basics

Obviously, you cannot perform reflexology without any first-hand knowledge on how it works and what are the key meridians or pressure points you need to target.

Read up first on the basic meridians found in feet, and what parts of the body are those meridians targeting.

Know Your Target

From what you have learned from the basics, know which part of the body you are targeting by using reflexology techniques. Each meridian in the feet can correspond to an organ like the kidney or liver.

Do the Whole Treatment

In foot reflexology, even if you are aiming for a specific part of the body or meridian to use as a gateway for treatment, do not forget to touch upon the other meridians to ensure a well-balanced reflexology session and health.

Relax Yourself

Whether you are your own reflexology patient

or you are doing this for another person, both of you should try to relax. Wear comfortable clothes and perform the therapy on a comfortable space, preferably a soft surface.

Apply Pressure Gently

Remember to apply pressure on the meridians gently. It takes not only knowledge but practice to master the techniques of foot reflexology. Remember that this is like a massage but greater – you are targeting parts of the body using the meridians on the feet.

Be Mindful

If you are doing reflexology for your partner or

someone else, always ask if he or she is alright with the pressure or if it hurts. Take note that a person may have a weaker pain tolerance level if he or she is sick (especially those who have fever or muscle pains) so be wary of this.

You should also consider not doing reflexology sessions for someone who's overslept for a long time.

Creams and Oils

Foot reflexology may sometimes be used with creams and oils, especially for couples who use it as a sensual activity that strengthens their husband-and-wife relationship.

However, they are best used after the session and not on the actual treatment because they can make meridian pressure application a bit more difficult due to the slippery texture.

Use Blankets

Since you can only work on one foot at a given time, you should prepare a blanket or towel to cover the other foot and keep it warm.

Rehydrate after a Reflexology Session

Drink a lot of water after the reflexology session to replenish. Since foot reflexology can speed up and improve our body's natural circulation, rehydration is important.

DIY Foot Massage Techniques

There are the specific massaging techniques you can use for different instances, such as stress-relieving or reducing pain:

Head and Neck

If you are experiencing headache, apply pressure on the joints of your toes, because they correspond to your neck. Repeat until the head and neck pressure disappears.

Toe Rotation

Rotating the toes help relieve headaches as well and strengthen bones. Start with the big toes first and work your way to the smallest.

Foot Instep

The instep is the middle part under your feet. In foot reflexology, applying pressure to the instep can relieve stomach upsets and any abdominal pains.

Relieve Insomnia

For those who are having problems in sleeping or insomnia, reflexology can help you by the following pressure points on your feet: back of the toes, outer edges, balls of the feet and the instep. By stimulating the said parts, you can help reduce stress and sleep better.

Relieve the Chest Areas

By stimulating the ball part of your feet, you can help relieve any pain in the chest area, such as the lungs, heart, chest, airways, thymus gland, shoulders and other important organs that foot reflexology can target.

Relax Arms and Legs

Using significant amount of pressure on the reflex points on the feet edges, you can help reduce tension and stress on your arms and legs.

Talcum or Baby Powder

While doing a reflexology session for yourself or another person, the use of talcum or baby powder makes it easier to apply pressure on meridians or reflex points. It also allows your hands to move freely without the slippery feel. Choosing a fragrant powder will best stimulate the mood.

Length of Session

The length of a session varies differently for people. However, on a normal foot reflexology session, 45 minutes should be enough.

However, do not go for more than 30 minutes

if you or your partner is sick, very young or an elderly due to their lower tolerances for pain. It may also depend on the size of the person's hands and feet.

Having a Session Partner is a Good Thing

Partner sessions are quite beneficial. Unless you are living alone or currently have no one to bother with your reflexology session, you can call up someone close to join and help out.

This will help you relax even more and ease the pain in your foot reflexology session, since you are not the one doing the pressure.

Watch for Post-Session Responses

Because not all of us have the same tolerance levels for pain and body structure, some people may experience post-session symptoms like coughing, decrease in energy, spasms, exhaustion and others. Therefore, it is important to immediately drink lots of water after a session.

Diabetic Warnings

Diabetic people who undergo reflexology should check their blood sugar levels before and after due to the body's sudden changes after the session.

Foot Massage For Common Problems

The world is a very busy place and our bodies are always susceptible to breakdowns when overused without proper rest or relaxation techniques. Like machines that get worn out after years of being used in the industry, our body works the same way.

If we don't relax ourselves and relieve the pain and stress, we might end up in a worst-case scenario, so it's an important aspect of life to do a massage once in a while.

Our feet are among the most sensitive parts of our body and in this book, we are going to enumerate different types of foot massages.

Reflexology Massage

This is an area-based massage technique on the foot, which divides it into several channels called meridians. These meridians can connect to different parts of the body like the liver, spleen, gallbladder, urinary bladder, stomach and kidneys.

Massaging and applying pressure on the foot using reflexology techniques can help alleviate stress, tension and ease the pain of certain illnesses, diseases and sickness, or even simple headaches. It may also reduce the likelihood of mental breakdowns, anxiety disorders and even depression.

Sports or Athlete Massage

As the name implies, this type of foot therapy is mostly used for athletes. Foot massages like this can help ease the pain of injuries, muscle strains and the like, and makes the use of different massaging techniques done before and after any sporting event.

It is also an aid for people who are having trouble with mobility (walking or running).

Hot Stone Massage

This massaging technique makes use of heated stones that are placed around a patient's feet to help relieve muscle strain. It is also a gentler and lighter massage which helps balance the body's energy. Some therapists may also apply pressure using the stones in hand.

Swedish Massage

This is one of the foot massages that are most commonly used at spas and treatment centers. It makes the use of various rhythmic techniques of stroking such as Friction, Petrissage, Tapotement and Effleurage.

The Swedish massage is said to bring up energy, invigoration, relaxation and a refreshing feeling to the patient. It relives muscles from too much tension and stress and is mostly used for people who are having problems with their joints or injuries.

Deep Tissue Massage

While this type of massage is less rhythmic and a bit slower, it can help repair, as the name implies, tissue injuries. It's one of the most common foot massages that help alleviate ailments in the limbs, stiff joints, and other muscle strains.

It works by applying pressure on some parts of the legs and joints to help soothe the patient's muscles and tissues.

Neuromuscular Therapy

Much like deep tissue massage, the neuromuscular therapy works by targeting different causes of pain.

Its main purpose is to increase and improve blood circulation throughout the body and strengthen the muscular system as well as the nervous system. It requires targeting the soft tissues of the body through the foot's instep.

Foot Massage Techniques For Common Problems

Along with the different types of foot massages, there are also individual techniques usually applied onto these types.

Stroking Method

Stroking is one of the most common methods of massaging the feet, starting from the toes all the way to the ankle.

Ankle Rotation Method

This technique is used to remove stiffness and tension of the ankle and feet joints. To do this, gently turn the ball of your foot 3 to 5 times on both directions (clockwise and counterclockwise), supported by a hand under the heel.

Toe Rotation Method

Start from the big toes to the small ones. One of the best and commonly-used techniques when implementing foot massages, toe rotation can help relieve headaches and strengthen bones.

Warm Up with Oils or Lotions

Before and after you do meridian-based massage pressure like in reflexology, you can warm up using essential oils and lotions that help revitalize the skin. This technique can also improve blood circulation.

First, apply and rub some of the oil or lotion on your hands. Afterwards, start rubbing from the toes all the way to the ankle.

Kneading Method

The kneading method focuses on the heel of the foot. Using a clench fist, gently press or knead the feet's soles.

Press the Arch Method

Many foot massages employ the press the arch method. Support your ankle and heel with one hand and rub the arch of the foot using your other hand's palm to about five times. Set the pressure level to normal and don't exert too much.

Conclusion

There are a lot of healthy benefits when you massage the feet, be it your own or another person's.

First of all, it helps in blood circulation and also body balance. It can target specific ailments in our body and help in the maintenance of internal organs by using the different techniques in foot massages.

It may also help in lowering blood pressure, detoxifying the body, improved immune system and relief from stress, anxiety disorders and depression after a long day's work.

Important Warning

Even though massaging the foot can have great health benefits for our body, we must also take note of different risk factors.

For instance, pregnant women, the elderly, young people and sick people need special types of massages or else something wrong can happen.

Pregnant women may labor early if the wrong part was massaged. Sick people, the elderly and young people have a lower tolerance for pain and pressure, so foot massages should not exceed 30 minutes for them.

People who suffer wounds should also be taken into consideration to avoid further excessive bleeding.

Remember that even if you do learn how to massage your own feet using the different types and techniques, it is still the best idea to consult a therapist with license and proper training.

This is to ensure that the pressure points are more accurate and they can address your body's specific needs through a well-applied and relaxing foot therapy.

More Books By James Heath

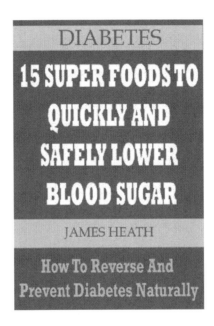

Introduction

With over 382 million people suffering from diabetes worldwide, it simply seems impossible to overlook the importance of learning ways to cope with this condition. In fact, it is expected that by 2035, around 592 million individuals will be affected by this disease.

To add to our worries, around 316 million people currently have high chances of developing type II diabetes, with around half of all people with the disease remaining undiagnosed at the global level.

Considering these statistics, you would definitely want to get your hands on reliable information that could help you and your loved ones cope with diabetes, particularly type II diabetes, which we all are at risk of developing at some point in our lives.

The basic difference between Type I and Type II diabetes is that people suffering from the former have a complete lack of insulin whereas for those with type II diabetes, there is too little insulin in the body, or the body can't use the available insulin effectively.

According to health experts, the most important factor in controlling, and often reversing type II diabetes is to eat the right foods.

And, you don't need my advice to understand that. Talk to your doctor or simply Google this topic, and you'll know what role your diet plays in helping you cope with, control, and prevent type II diabetes.

Yes, you read it right! Type II diabetes can be prevented, controlled, and even reversed, if you choose foods that not only help in stabilizing your blood sugar but that also play an important role in promoting weight loss.

In this book, I've talked about 15 super foods that can help lower your blood sugar levels so that you can live a healthier, longer life.

Almonds- Maintain Your Blood Glucose Levels

Whether it is the high concentration of monounsaturated fats that can reduce your chances of developing heart disease or the Vitamin E present in this super food, almonds are the best friends for people with type II diabetes.

They are rich in magnesium, which plays an important role in improving the flow of nutrient, blood as well as oxygen throughout the body. Moreover, almonds contain potassium, which serves as an electrolyte for muscle contraction as well as for nerve transmission in your body.

For people with diabetes, eating almonds means reduced after-meal blood glucose and insulin levels. In fact, if you are coupling almonds with a high glycemic index food, you are actually reducing your meal's glycemic index while decreasing after-meal blood sugar levels.

According to a study, if you choose to replace 20 percent of dietary calories with almonds, you will end up with better markers of insulin sensitivity as well as improved cholesterol levels.

So, try adding a handful of almonds to your fruity snacks or top salads with toasted almonds to reap the benefits of this delicious nut!

Click Here To Read More!

Or Go To: http://amzn.to/1EnoAoC

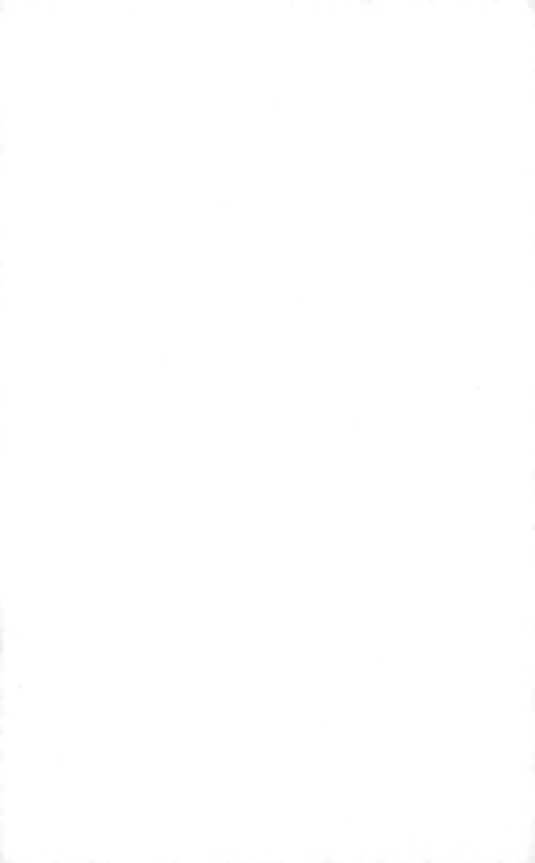

Made in the USA
Lexington, KY
27 January 2015